HOMOEOPATHIC MEDICINE

HARRIS L. COULTER, Ph.D.

Formur, Inc.—St. Louis
Publishers

Library of Congress
Catalogue Card Number
74-190020

Copyright 1972 by

American Foundation for Homoeopathy

Copyright 1975 by

American Foundation for
Homoeopathy and Formur, Inc.

Second printing since 1975

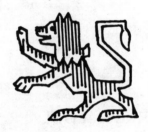

Published under license by FORMUR, INC.
PUBLISHERS, 4200 Laclede Avenue, St. Louis,
Missouri 63108 in conjunction with the National
Center for Homoeopathy, 6231 Leesburg Pike,
Falls Church, Virginia 22044

ISBN 0-89378-072-3

PRINTED IN THE UNITED STATES OF AMERICA

CONTENTS

HOMOEOPATHIC MEDICINE

Homoeopathy is a system of drug therapy, a set of rules governing the administration of drugs to sick people. These rules enable the physician to understand the patient's illness and to prescribe the drug which will act curatively.

The homoeopathic rules were developed by following the procedures of scientific method, and homoeopathy is, therefore, a scientific form of drug therapeutics. Since a scientific truth is universal, homoeopathy claims universality for its rules of drug use and, except in comparatively few instances, does not view the prescribing of drugs on other principles as beneficial to the patient.

This essay sets forth the homoeopathic rules and indicates why they are scientific, why homoeopathic medicine is "scientific medicine." An exposition of these rules necessarily involves reference to the prevailing orthodox system of medical practice (which in the homoeopathic literature is called "allopathy"), and we will proceed essentially by way of a contrast between the homoeopathic rules and principles and those accepted in the allopathic practice of medicine.

I. ASSUMPTIONS ABOUT HEALTH AND DISEASE

Any system of medical practice takes its origin in a set of assumptions about health and disease. Sometimes these assumptions are conscious and explicit. More often they are unconscious; the practitioner is unaware of them. The homoeopathic and allopathic approaches to therapeutics are based on sets of assumptions about disease, health, and the curative process. Furthermore, these two sets of assumptions are opposed to one another in many important respects. The different therapeutic procedures employed by homoeopathy and allopathy originate in different interpretations of observed physiological and pathological processes.

From Hahnemann[1] onwards, the homoeopathic physicians have characterized the processes of health and disease in vitalistic terms. They have talked of a "vital force", "power of recovery", or "natural force" in the body—a force which reacts to external stimuli. This reactive power is manifested in the symptoms of disease, just as it also makes its presence felt in the rhythmic alterations of the body's functions in health; the alternation of

---

[1]Samuel Hahnemann (1755–1843), the founder of the homoeopathic system of medicine.

sleep and wakefulness, the menstrual function in women, etc. Disease symptoms represent the form taken by this power when reacting to a morbific stimulus in the internal or external environment.

The vitalistic assumption is of primordial importance for homoeopathic therapeutics, since it imposes a particular interpretation of the symptom. Regardless of how disagreeable or even painful it may be, the symptom is still the visible manifestation of the organism's reactive power. And since this reactive power always strives for cure, for harmony in the functioning of the organism, and always strives to adjust the balance between the body and its environment, the symptoms are not the signs of a morbific, but of a curative, process. They point out to the physician the route taken by the body in coping with some particular stress; hence they are the best guides to treatment. Since the body's reactive force endeavors to cope with a given stress by producing *a particular set of symptoms*, the physician's duty is to promote the development of this very set of symptoms. The curative medicine is the one which supports and stimulates the organism's incipient and inchoate healing effort.

Experience has shown that symptoms appear and disappear in a definite order when the sick person is treated in accordance with the homoeopathic rules.

In the first place, they disappear in the reverse order of their appearance, the chronologically most recent being replaced by those of the earlier stages of the disease. A corollary is that some phase of a disease which has been suppressed by incorrect treatment at an earlier stage of the patient's life will reappear when the correct medicine is administered and can then be "cured".[2]

[2]We are compelled to use the words, "cure" and "recovery", because there are no convenient substitutes. The reader will be aware that even in homoeopathic practice the concepts are ambiguous, involving the complexities of Hering's Law and of Hahnemann's theory of chronic disease.

4

In the second place, the symptoms will move from the more vital organs to the less vital and from the interior of the body toward the skin.

In the third place, the symptoms will move from the top of the body downward—disappearing first from the head, then from the torso, and then from the extremities, proceeding from the shoulders to the elbow, wrist, and hand, or from the thigh to the knee, ankle, and foot.

These rules are known in homoeopathy as Hering's Law, in honor of Constantine Hering (1800–1880), the Father of American Homoeopathy, who discerned them and thus made the only major addition to Hahnemann's initial system. Hering's Law can be illustrated as follows: (1) an arthritis which started in the right hip, and then moved to the left, should disappear first from the left hip and then from the right; (2) when a case of arthritis complicated with endocarditis is treated correctly, the heart symptoms are the first to disappear, being followed by the symptoms of the upper joints and finally by those of the lower joints; (3) correct treatment of a female patient with uterine complaints caused these symptoms to be replaced by symptoms of a scarlet fever which had been suppressed by incorrect treatment thirty years before; cure was complete when the appropriate remedy was administered for the newly appearing scarlet-fever symptoms.

Homoeopathy stresses the importance of the body's natural discharges—urine, stool, menses, and especially skin eruptions. The organism's natural tendency in health is to rid itself of waste substances through these natural outlets, and a similar process is at work in disease. The suppression of natural secretions and eruptions can give rise to serious systemic disorders. Skin eruptions are the manifestation of nature's effort to throw off some internal toxin or waste matter. The suppression of eczema by local applications has been known to produce colitis, asthma, and bronchitis. The suppression of syphilitic and gon-norrhoeal skin symptoms can give rise to a myriad of chronic manifestations. Medicines must strengthen and intensify the processes adopted by the organism to cope with morbific stimuli and must never counteract these processes.

Another corollary of Hering's Law is homoeopathy's stress on the significance of mental symptoms for treatment. All somatic diseases manifest mental symptoms in addition to the physical ones, and the homoeopathic practitioner views these symptoms as profoundly important. Why? Because they are at the same time the symptoms of a vital organ, of the interior of the body, and of the highest part of the body. In treatment these should be the first to disappear, and if the symptoms do move from the mind to the less vital parts, the physician knows that he is employing the correct medicine.

In other words, homoeopathy denies any inherent distinction between physical and mental illness. Physical illnesses have a mental aspect, and mental illnesses have a physical aspect. The physician should understand the significance of both physical and mental symptoms, and of their interaction. The prescription of drugs in homoeopathy is based upon a consideration of both types of symptoms, and these physicians were treating some mental illnesses successfully with drugs 150 years ago.

If we now attempt to elucidate the assumptions about health and disease current in orthodox practice, we find ourselves in a quandary, because modern allopathic medicine does not admit to any explicit set of assumptions in this area. A writer has observed that modern medicine shies away from any general theory of the organism, of health, and of disease.[3] A little thought, however,

[3]Ian Stevenson, M.D., "Why Medicine Is Not A Science", *Harpers*, April, 1949, pp. 36–39.

will disclose two important tenets of modern allopathic medicine. One relates to the symptom—allopathic medicine does not generally regard the symptom as a sign of the body's reaction to morbific environmental stimuli, but rather as a wound inflicted upon the body by morbific stimuli. Far from considering that the body reacts dynamically to external stimuli, allopathic medicine tends to view the body as the passive recipient of blows delivered from the outside.

The other major tenet of allopathic medicine is the "disease entity" or "clinical entity." Knud Faber has written that the physician "cannot live, cannot speak, cannot act, without [it]."[4] What is the meaning of the disease entity? It means that the symptoms—the "wounds which the environment inflicts upon the body"—can be grouped into typical patterns and viewed as discrete diseases. Thus allopathic medicine operates with a relatively static group of discrete "diseases." This is to be contrasted with the dynamic doctrine of disease categories employed in homoeopathy.[5]

While, in allopathic medicine, the persons within each disease category will differ from one another in certain respects, for purposes of diagnosis and treatment the common elements are considered to be of greater significance than the points of difference. The physician bases his treatment upon the elements which the patients within each category possess in common.

These common elements may be bacterial, symptomatic, morphological, or other. What interests us is the logical idea that these common elements are the phenomena of primary interest to the physician.

This idea, which has an ancient lineage and is found in

[4]Knud Faber, "Nosography In Modern Internal Medicine", *Annals of Medical History* IV (1922), p. 63.
[5]Discussed on pages 20, 25, 30–32, 38.

several of the Hippocratic writings, has at times given rise to the extreme position that the disease is a metaphysical entity. As Sir Clifford Allbutt has written: "It was born to signify that reality of substance which was once supposed to underlie abstract names, and in these ontological circles it has moved ever since."[6] Since his time, about 70 years ago, all prominent spokesmen for allopathic medicine have rejected this understanding of the disease entity. But no attempt has since been made to create a precise theoretical definition of the disease entity. Furthermore, physicians often seem to adhere to the idea that the disease is, in fact, an entity in the ontological sense denounced by Allbutt. The very word, "entity", is used in medical writing. This aberration is, of course, favored by the absence of an accepted theory of the disease entity.

There is a psychological connection between the disease-entity concept and the view that the symptom is a lesion inflicted by a morbific stimulus. The entity is built up from the prominent or striking symptoms; attention is directed to these symptoms, and it is thus natural to regard them as harmful manifestations. Fever is a good example. While the homoeopathic physician will regard fever as a benign symptom, reflecting the body's effort to overcome the morbific influence at work on the body, the orthodox physician will take the contrary view and administer medicines which lower the fever. (It is fair to note that the contrary interpretation of fever is also occasionally given in the allopathic medical writings, but then how is the physician to distinguish the benign fever from the one which is harmful?) Many of the medicines used in allopathic practice aim to oppose or counteract one or several prominent disease symptoms.

[6]Quoted in Otto Guttentag, M.D., "On The Clinical Entity", *Annals of Internal Medicine* XXXI (1949), p. 488.

8

We may carry the analysis a step further and note that the allopathic physician's attitude toward the symptom determines his attitude toward the "vital force." He cannot admit the existence of such a force in the body and at the same time administer medicines which counteract or suppress the symptoms which are the very manifestations of this force. Hence he instinctively rejects the vital-force doctrine.

Thus the homoeopath and the regular physician start off with divergent interpretations of the symptom. The concept of the vital force is of considerable moment for the day-to-day practice of medicine in the homoeopathic school, and its rejection by medical orthodoxy has a similarly pronounced effect on the practice of allopathic medicine.

This concept is significant in yet another way. Its acceptance by homoeopathy symbolizes the deeply held conviction of this school that the internal processes of the organism are (1) extremely complex and not to be wholly comprehended by the physician—so that therapy may not be based upon this assumed knowledge, and (2) linked to one another in such a way as to make all parts of the organism interdependent—so that any attempt at treatment must be treatment of the whole patient, treatment which is proportioned to all parts and systems of the body and not merely treatment of one organ or part of the body.

Thus the reader should not be misled by the homoeopathic use of the expression, "vital force." It in no way implies a "mystical", "eighteenth-century", or "unscientific" approach to medicine. It does not imply any particular view of the essential nature of the organism but has a practical meaning in compelling the physician: (1) to take a humble view of his own ability to penetrate intellectually into the human body, and (2) to bear in mind at all times that any treatment must be treatment of the whole body, the whole man.

In thus stressing the ultimate unknowability of the body's physiological and psychological processes, homoeopathy is in agreement with the most recent standpoint of theoretical physics and of Jungian analytical psychology, both of which accept the ultimate indeterminacy of the phenomena investigated and call for a symbolic, "as if", approach to their understanding.

That the holism of the homoeopathic view of the organism is not without relevance for modern medicine is clear to anyone who has followed the discussion—during the last twenty years or so—of the typical defect of modern orthodox medical practice, which is precisely that the physician fails to pay sufficient attention to the wholeness of the patient, fails to adjust his treatment to the whole man. There is even a "crisis in medical education"—meaning that the medical student fails to acquire a feeling for the wholeness of the patient—and programs are elaborated for adjusting the medical school curriculum in such a way as to impart this feeling to the student.

Such efforts cannot be successful, however, in the absence of an integrated theory of the whole man. The mere reorganization of the curriculum, exhortations to the medical student to pay more attention to the psychological, sociological, or epidemiological background of his patients, can have no effect unless integrated into a therapeutic theory whose point of departure is a theory of the whole organism.

Allopathic medicine, however, does not possess such a theory and manifests no interest in acquiring one. The closest it comes to a basic theoretical tenet is its concept of the disease entity.

In contrast, homoeopathy does possess a precise theory of the organism—one which enables its practitioners to comprehend the significance of individual symptoms as well as the dynamic interaction among symptoms in health and disease. When asked how he can be sure that this theory is valid, the homoeopathic physician will respond that it has served for 150 years as the basis for the successful homoeopathic treatment of disease and the preservation of health. And if the homoeopathic physician *can* cure his patients consistently and methodically on the basis of this theory, this set of assumptions, who is to say that it is wrong? Practice is the only test. No one is justified in attacking the assumption of the vital force, and its theoretical and practical corollaries, unless he can produce a better theory—one which yields better practical results.

II. EPISTEMOLOGICAL ASSUMPTIONS:

The Physician's Knowledge of the Organism
and the Effects of Medicines

The physician's first task is to know what his patient is suffering from. His second task is to cure this patient. Thus he first needs a key to understanding the organism and, secondly, a key to the effects of medicines.

Let us first take up the problem of ascertaining what ails the patient. The physician has two sources of knowledge. The first is sense-perception, defined as including (1) that which is perceivable by the physician and (2) that which is perceivable by the patient and which can be elicited from him by careful questioning. The second source of knowledge—defined, in allopathic medicine, as "objective"—includes the various tests which have been devised for measuring the chemical composition of the blood and the other bodily fluids, for examining and analyzing the structure of the tissues, for measuring blood pressure, for recording brain waves, and the like. Generally speaking, these data are not directly sense-perceptible, and this knowledge is not symptomatic knowledge. It is knowledge of the physiological and pathological changes occurring in the body during disease.

The homoeopathic and orthodox physicians take opposed views of the nature and importance of these two kinds of knowledge. The former attribute prime importance to sensory knowledge of the patient's symptoms and secondary importance to the so-called "objective" disease parameters. With the latter, this emphasis is reversed. Allopathic physicians attribute greater importance to the "objective" information and less to the "subjective" symptoms.

The difference stems from homoeopathy's orientation toward the dynamic and changeable vital force, as opposed to allopathic medicine's concentration on the static disease entity. This initial difference in approach leads to different views of the relative importance of the symptoms and the "objective" pathological or physiological data.

Homoeopathy holds that the disease process first affects the vital force, where its presence is manifested by a change in the patient's general well-being—before any "objective" changes can be noted in the patient's fluids or tissues. These pathological changes are the *result* of the alteration in the vital principle and not its *cause*. The initial morbid changes in the state of the vital force are, therefore, expressed only as symptoms. Symptoms are chronologically prior to pathology. For this reason they are also prior in importance. The ongoing pathological changes are, at all stages, preceded by symptomatic changes. Attention to these symptomatic changes will enable the physician to forestall the pathological deterioration.

The homoeopathic physician of today will conduct the same chemical, microscopic, and other tests of the patient's tissues and fluids as are done by the allopathic physician, but he is always aware that they yield knowledge of the *consequences* of pathological alterations in

14

the vital force. Tissue and fluid changes are chronologically posterior to the alterations in the vital force itself, and knowledge of these changes must therefore be of secondary importance for treatment.

The alterations in the vital force are to be perceived only by a most careful and exhaustive analysis of symptoms. Hahnemann exhorted the physician to observe with extreme care everything that was to be seen with the eyes or perceived in any way by the other senses. Above all, the physician was to question the patient minutely about his perceptions and sensations. If the physician's interrogation and observation of the patient were sufficiently thorough, as Hahnemann thought, he would have all the information needed to effect a cure in those cases where cure is possible.

> "The internal essential nature of every malady, of every individual case of disease, as far as it is necessary for us to know it, for the purpose of curing it, expresses itself by the *symptoms*, as they present themselves to the investigations of the true observer in their whole extent, connection, and succession.
>
> When the physician has discovered all the observable symptoms of the disease that exist, he has discovered the disease itself, he has attained the complete conception of it requisite to enable him to effect a cure."[7]

Hahnemann had strong objections to the cursory and superficial way in which most physicians examined their patients and proposed a far more comprehensive technique for observing and registering these all-important indicators of disease.

> "For example, what is the character of his stools? How does he pass his water? How is it with his day and night sleep? What is the state of his disposition, his humor, his memory? How about

[7]Samuel Hahnemann, *Lesser Writings*, New York: William Radde, 1852, p. 443.

the thirst? What sort of taste has he in his mouth? What kinds of food and drink are most relished? What are most repugnant to him? Has each its full natural taste, or some other unusual taste? How does he feel after eating or drinking? Has he anything to tell about the head, the limbs, or the abdomen? . . . What did the patient vomit? Is the bad taste in his mouth putrid or bitter or sour, or what? Before or after eating or during the repast? At what period of the day was it worst? What is the taste of what is eructated? Does the urine only become turbid on standing, or is it turbid when first discharged? . . . Does he start during sleep? Does he lie only on his back, or on which side? Does he cover himself well up, or can he not bear the clothes on him? Does he easily awake, or does he sleep too soundly? How does he feel immediately after waking from sleep? How often does this or that symptom occur? What is the cause that produces it each time it occurs? Does it come on whilst sitting, lying, standing, or when in motion? Only when fasting? . . . how the patient behaved during the visit—whether he was morose, quarrelsome, hasty, lachrymose, anxious, despairing, or sad, or hopeful, calm, etc. Whether he was in a drowsy state or in any way dull of comprehension; whether he spoke hoarsely or in a low tone or incoherently, or how otherwise did he talk? What was the color of his face and eyes, and of his skin generally? What degree of liveliness and power was there in his expression and eyes? What was the state of his tongue, his breathing, the smell from his mouth, and his hearing? Were his pupils dilated or contracted? How rapidly and to what extent did they alter in the dark and in the light? What was the character of the pulse? What the condition of the abdomen? How moist or hot, how cold or dry to the touch, was the skin of this or that part, or generally? Whether he lay with head thrown back with mouth half or fully open, with the arms placed above the head, on his back, or in what other position? What effort did he make to raise himself? And anything else in him that may strike the physician as being remarkable."[8]

Thus the homoeopath must record a long list of symptoms, including many which would be ignored by the

[8]Samuel Hahnemann, *The Organon of Medicine*, Sixth Edition. Translated with Preface by William Boericke, M.D., and Introduction by James Krauss, M.D. Calcutta: Roysingh and Co., 1962. Notes to Sections 88–90.

orthodox physician. He must pay special attention to the "modalities": Is the particular symptom aggravated or relieved by heat, cold, motion, rest, noise, quiet, wetness, dryness, and changes in the weather? In the homoeopathic view all these symptoms are important in giving the detailed knowledge of the patient's state which the physician must have if he is to effect a cure. These changes in the symptoms produced by different environmental conditions are often the key to the correct medicine.

Hahnemann categorically denied the value of pathological theory for the cure of disease. This was his natural reaction to the overweening speculation practised in the orthodox medicine of his day. Being a religious man, Hahnemann decided that God must have given the physician some better alternative than theorizing, and this alternative was reliance on the data presented to the senses. Hence he exhorted the physician to ignore internal pathology and rely entirely on sense-perceptible symptoms.

Today pathological theory has made considerable advances, and its measurement techniques are more varied and precise than in Hahnemann's times. The homoeopathic physician is entitled to depart from Hahnemann's strict rejection of pathology and to rely somewhat on this knowledge. But pathological knowledge still remains unstable—as is seen from the continuing flux and change in pathological theories—while the symptom-patterns of disease are essentially the same today as in Hahnemann's times. Where they have changed, these changes can be noted accurately by the observant physician. Symptomatic knowledge, therefore, remains more reliable than pathological knowledge, and homoeopathy still insists on the priority of the symptoms over "objective" pathological parameters.

After all, there is no *a priori* reason to assume that diseases are not capable of being accurately measured in terms of their symptoms. While only a highly skilled physician can elicit a true and complete disease description by this method, the method itself is intrinsically accurate. To seek a greater degree of precision in the measurement of vital phenomena would be an error. Aristotle has noted that the educated man does not seek greater precision than is inherent in the subject-matter. The homoeopaths feel that the so-called objective measurement techniques of orthodox medicine all too often yield a spurious precision—highly refined data which have no precise meaning, no precise therapeutic application.

The allopathic physician takes the contrary view, feeling that these parameters are more reliable guides to treatment precisely because they are "objective", while the "subjective" symptoms are too ephemeral and unstable to be reliable. While he does note the symptoms generally, he does not go into them in the exhaustive way urged by Hahnemann, and the diagnosis will always rely more heavily upon the "objective" parameters than upon the "unstable" or "evanescent" symptoms.

The attempt to balance symptoms and "objective" findings places this physician in a dilemma. Symptoms are very numerous, as homoeopathic experience indicates. But the orthodox physician is not interested in *all* the patient's symptoms, only in the "important" ones, the ones which characterize unambiguously the presence of some typical disease process. But the "importance" of a given symptom is, of course, related to the diagnosis which is ultimately accepted. The physician may simply discard all the symptoms which do not fit the diagnosis, ascribing them to the patient's tendency to neurosis or hypochondria. Or he may retain some of them on the ground that the case is "atypical". What is important is that he does not base the diagnosis on all possible observable symptoms but arbitrarily accepts some of them and discards others. Hahnemann remarked in this connection:

> " 'What do we care,' say the medical teachers and their books, 'what do we care about the presence of many other diverse symptoms that are observable in the case of disease before us, or the absence of those that are wanting? The physician should pay no attention to such empirical trifles; his practical tact, the penetrating glance of his mental eye into the hidden nature of the malady, enables him to determine at the very first sight of the patient what is the matter with him, what pathological form of the disease he has to do with, and what name he has to give it . . .' "[9]

Hahnemann felt that therapy should not be based upon a conclusion about the internal state of the organism, because this knowledge is unstable and arbitrary—reflecting an arbitrary selection among the symptoms. The allopathic physician cannot take into account all the symptoms presented by the patient because he would not know what to do with them anyway. Many cannot be referred to some accepted pathological process. But these may be the very ones which best define the illness from which the patient is suffering. Who is to say that they are unimportant?

For the time being, we may note that allopathic medicine is ambiguous in its attitude toward the symptoms. This question will be discussed further below.[10]

Here it may only be suggested that an important reason for allopathic medicine's insistence upon "objective" data as the basis for diagnosis is that reliance upon sense-perception alone—upon the symptoms—leads to a tre-

[9]Hahnemann, *Lesser Writings*, p. 714.
[10]See pages 27, 30, 58.

mendous proliferation of possible disease states. Any physician knows that the variety among patients is inexhaustible. If symptoms alone are to be the guide, where is the physician to find a principle for grouping the individual cases into recognizable categories?

Homoeopathy was confronted with this same problem. Hahnemann refused to group patients according to their pathological indications. In his view this blurred the small but significant differences among patients. He maintained that each case is unique and that the physician's task is not to ignore this uniqueness but to find some *methodical* way of adapting treatment to the specific needs of each patient.

The solution was found through a complete reorientation of medical thought. Hahnemann decided that diseased states must be classified—not in terms of their prominent symptoms—but in terms of the *medicines which cure them.*

This introduces our discussion of the physician's second task, as defined above—how to find a reliable guide to the operations of medicines.

Here the same contrast between the homoeopathic and allopathic approaches may be noted as held for their differing approaches to diagnosis. Homoeopathy maintains that, for evaluating the mode of action of a medicinal drug, sensory perception of the symptoms is a more reliable guide than the "objective" measurement of physiological parameters. The methodological differences to which this leads will best be understood by first examining the techniques used today by orthodox medicine to ascertain the therapeutic powers of medicines.

These techniques are numerous, but their underlying principle is the same: given the existence of a such-and-such a disease entity, find a medicine whose mode of

action will oppose or counteract the fundamental processes at work in the disease.

Allopathic medicine aims to develop a theory of drug
action which it combines with a theory of the disease
entity.

It is quite difficult in contemporary allopathic medicine
to determine which new medicine will be effective in a
given "disease". There is a body of knowledge known as
pharmacological theory, but this theory is still too crude
to give *a priori* information about the action of drugs.
"There does not exist any sound theoretical basis on
which to build a rational approach to the search for really
new types of drugs."[11] "There are few drugs, if any, for
which we know the basic mechanism of action."[12] "To
date, the subject of biochemorphology has advanced to
the point where intelligent guesses may be made as to the
influence of alteration in structure on the activity of a
given molecule. However, prediction of usefulness and
safety on this basis is impossible."[13] The dependence of
biological performance on chemical and molecular structure is, in fact, so erratic that even changes in the manu-
facturing process will sometimes alter therapeutic action
in an unacceptable way and compel withdrawal of the
medicine from the market.

Consequently, pharmacological theory only offers suggested lines of research, and these suggestions must be
tested through trials on animals and ultimately on
humans. Medicines are tested for their toxicological
effect and their gross physiological effect on some organ

[11]Rene Dubos, in Paul Talalay, ed., *Drugs in our Society*, Baltimore: Johns
Hopkins, 1964, p. 37.

[12]Louis S. Goodman, in *ibid.*, p. 54.

[13]Victor A. Drill, Ph.D., M.D., *Pharmacology in Medicine*, New York: Mc-
Graw-Hill, 1954, p. 1/16.

or organ system in animals. For the actual therapeutic trial, it is necessary to gather together a group of persons suffering from the "same disease" and administer the medicine to them (following the accepted procedures for ensuring statistical validity of the results, eliminating observer bias, etc.), then subject the results to appropriate statistical analysis. If the patients in the group receiving the medicine seem to benefit from it, by comparison with those under traditional treatment or those receiving a placebo, and this benefit falls within the area of statistical significance, the medicine is viewed as possessing some therapeutic potential.

The methodological defects in this procedure will be discussed in more detail below. Here let us merely note that the procedure is subject to two major criticisms from the homoeopathic standpoint. The first is that the medicines are usually evaluated in terms of some "objectively" measurable parameter. But these "objective" phenomena are the effects of the changes which the drug has made in the pattern of the vital force. Hence it would be far better to measure the changes in the vital force rather than the mere consequences of such changes. The second is that this procedure is based upon the assumed existence of a disease entity—upon the assumed possibility of grouping cases in terms of their striking or common characteristics and ignoring the points of dissimilarity.

In his day, Hahnemann was confronted with the same problem, as the testing of medicines by his contemporaries was also premised upon the existence of the disease entity.The physician tried out new medicines on those of his patients whom he suspected of suffering from the disease for which the medicine was supposed to be beneficial. He reported the results, other physicians tried out the remedy, and it was subsequently either accepted or rejected by the profession as a whole.

Although vaunted on all sides as thoroughly "empirical", this drug-testing procedure was an unstable mixture of sensory symptomatic data and the measurements of pathological parameters. Hahnemann thought that this was imprecise and speculative. He objected, as homoeopathic physicians object today, that the disease descriptions were too imprecise and that the "disease entity" contains many quite dissimilar diseased states which should perhaps be treated by a number of different remedies.

As proof of his argument, he pointed out that the most acclaimed medicines often have a very short life expectancy, being denounced as regularly—after the profession has accumulated some years of experience with them—as they were praised upon their introduction.

Hahnemann was then faced with the problem of devising a substitute procedure for ascertaining the curative powers of medicines, one which would meet all the criteria which he had set himself:

1) The procedure must avoid recourse to the disease entity:

2) The procedure must be based primarily upon sensory data; just as physiological processes are best described by their sense-perceptible manifestations, the alterations in these processes caused by medicines are also best described in sensory terms.

Hahnemann's solution to this problem was his adoption of the Law of Similars as the foundation-stone of homoeopathic therapeutics. The Law of Similars has figured in medical history since the time of Hippocrates. While it has had different meanings at different times, in Hahnemann's formulation it meant that each medicinal substance will cure the patient whose total set of symptoms corresponds precisely to the set of symptoms produced by the same substance when administered to a healthy person.

Hence the name, homoeopathy, from the Greek: *homoion pathos*, meaning "similar disease."

If a healthy person takes any drug or medicinal substance on a regular basis for several days or weeks, he will come to manifest a set of symptoms which are peculiar to the particular drug or substance.[14] In homoeopathic philosophy, this procedure is known as "proving" the medicine (from the German: *Pruefung*, meaning "test" or "trial"). Calomel by its physiological action produces diarrhoea, frequent bloody and mucous stools, increased secretion of bile, and salivation. When a case of disease is characterized by these symptoms, very small doses of calomel (*Mercurius dulcis*) will be curative. *Belladonna* is indicated homoeopathically when the patient presents dilated pupils, violent congestion of blood to the head with throbbing headache, high fever with hot red skin, cerebral excitement, dryness of mouth and throat, muscular twitchings (the symptoms frequently encountered in scarlet fever). Any physician will recognize these symptoms as the well-known toxic effects of *Belladonna*.

Thus, when the homoeopathic physician has a complete and exhaustive listing of the patient's symptoms, he compares this with the listings of symptoms in the homoeopathic books of provings. When there is precise correspondence between the patient's symptoms and the symptoms of some particular medicine, as listed in the books of provings, this medicine will act curatively.

It will be seen that Hahnemann's assumption that the symptom is a benign manifestation is perfectly adapted to therapy based upon the Law of Similars. If the symp-

---

[14]Persons who are particularly sensitive to a given drug will manifest the drug's symptomatology to a more marked degree. Those who are less sensitive will yield a less striking symptom picture.

tom is recognized as the expression of the organism's effort to counteract morbific stimuli and to rid itself of disease, the medicine which stimulates the organism in precisely this direction is the one which will act curatively. Thus in homoeopathy the symptoms, which are the sense-perceptible evidence of the disease process, are at the same time sufficient to characterize the effects of medicines upon the organism. The disease process and the operations of medicines are described by sensory phenomena.

By the same token it is seen that the Law of Similars yields the basis for the homoeopathic classification of diseases. The traditional disease categories are largely rejected, and these physicians, if pressed, will only say that the patient has a *Sulphur* disease, *Belladonna* disease, *Cantharis* disease, or the like.[15] From the therapeutic viewpoint, what more useful criterion of disease classification could be desired than the medicine which acts curatively?

---

[15]James Tyler Kent, the foremost American homoeopath of an earlier generation, tells the story of an Irishman who came into the clinic one day, gave his symptoms, and then wanted to know what he had. "The physician answered, 'Why you have *Nux Vomica*,' that being his remedy. Whereupon the old man said, 'Well, I did think I had some wonderful disease or other' . . . " (Kent, *Lectures on Homoeopathic Philosophy*, Indian Edition, Calcutta: Sett Day & Co., 1961.)

III. THE HOMOEOPATHIC THERAPEUTIC METHOD

Hahnemann aimed to elaborate a therapeutic method which would enable the physician to account for the minute distinctions among patients and among remedies. The thrust of this system was to be contrary to that of orthodox medicine—which often classifies patients under the same diagnosis despite quite significant symptomatic differences and which also fails to distinguish among medicines with approximately similar modes of action.

Hahnemann presented his system in the form of the three rules: 1) prescription of the drug according to the Law of Similars, 2) the minimum dose, and 3) the single remedy.

1.) *The Law of Similars.* The homoeopathic physician must select his remedy on the basis of the *totality* of the patient's symptoms. This leads to a further distinction between the homoeopathic and the allopathic views of the relative importance of symptoms. While orthodox medicine stresses the obvious and striking symptoms, those which cause the patient the greatest unease, homoeopathy views these as of lesser importance than the symptoms peculiar to the given patient—the ones which he manifests and which another patient would not manifest under the same circumstances. As Hahnemann wrote, "the more common and undefined symptoms: loss of appetite, headache, debility, restless sleep, discomfort, and so forth, demand but little attention when of that vague and undefined character, if they cannot be more accurately described, as symptoms of such a common nature are observed in almost every disease and from almost every drug."[16] "The most singular, most uncommon signs furnish the characteristic, distinctive, and peculiar features."[17] "The more striking, singular, uncommon, and peculiar (characteristic) signs and symptoms of the case of disease are chiefly and most solely to be kept in view."[18]

The medicine which resembles the patient's syndrome in only its more common features will have little or no curative effect. The highly similar remedy, the *similimum*, derives its curative power from its close resemblance to the fleeting but strongly characteristic symptoms of the patient. Hahnemann, whose father wrote a treatise on portrait-painting, used the artist's language to express his idea of how the picture of the disease should be matched to the picture of the remedy:

"No portrait-painter was ever so careless as to pay no attention to the marked peculiarity in the features of the person he wished to make a likeness of, or to consider it sufficient to make any sort of a pair of round holes below the forehead by way of eyes, between them to draw a long-shaped thing directed downwards, always of the same shape, by way of a nose, and beneath this to put a slit going across the face, and should stand for the mouth of this or of any other person; no painter, I say, ever went about delineating human faces in such a rude and slovenly manner; no naturalist ever went to work in this fashion in describing any

[16]Hahnemann, *Organon*, Section 153.
[17]Hahnemann, *Lesser Writings*, pp. 181, 444.
[18]Hahnemann, *Organon*, Section 153.

natural production; such was never the way in which any zoologist, botanist, or mineralogist acted. It was only the semeiology of ordinary medicine that went to work in such a manner, when describing morbid phenomena."[19]

The key to the remedy is furnished by the small differences which distinguish one patient from another, one case of "pneumonia" or "scarlet fever" from another. These are the details which "individualize" the case, which reveal the peculiar features, the wholeness, of the disease and of the remedy. To ensure that these details were preserved in all their freshness and purity, Hahnemann urged the physician to take down the patient's symptoms in the *patient's own words* whenever possible. Homoeopathic experience has shown that the patient's own novel way of expressing his sensations is often paralleled precisely in the records of the provings, and these rare and peculiar symptoms are often of the greatest value to the physician.

Homoeopathic physicians since Hahnemann's time have made further study of the different grades of symptoms and of their relative importance. They have found that mental symptoms, when well defined, are usually the most useful. Then come the general symptoms: the patient's overall reaction to heat, cold, movement, foods, wet or dry weather, etc. Finally come the particular symptoms: those relating to a part of the body. In all three of these categories the symptoms which are absolutely dominant are the "strange, rare, and peculiar" symptoms which qualify the given patient and distinguish him from all others with similar mental, general, or particular symptoms.

The homoeopathic gradation of symptoms is a complex doctrine which cannot be elaborated in any detail here.

[19]Hahnemann, *Lesser Writings*, p. 727.

The reader is referred to the competent discussion of the subject by Margaret Tyler, M.D.[20]

The homoeopathic analysis of symptoms provides a sound method for "treating the patient and not the disease." This is an oft-mentioned desideratum in orthodox medicine but one which is difficult, if not impossible, to attain with a method based upon the concept of the disease entity. The disease entity, of necessity, directs the physician's attention away from the rare and peculiar symptoms (since they cannot usually be associated with any pathology) and toward the common symptoms of the various cases subsumed under a single disease name.

This attention to the common symptoms of disease is what makes orthodox medicine "scientific" in its own estimation. These physicians endeavor to treat the fever, the inflammation, the severe headache, the thirst, the restlessness, etc. which are striking features of very many different diseases. The homoeopath, on the contrary, denies the utility of these common symptoms precisely because they are common to so many diseases and so many cases of the same disease: he maintains that the scientific method is the one which enables the physician to take into account the minute but significant differences between one patient and another.

If patients are to be distinguished minutely from one another, it must also be possible to distinguish remedies in the same way. And just as the unusual symptoms are the key to the uniqueness of the particular patient, so these same symptoms in the provings are the key to the uniqueness of the particular remedy. Hahnemann's comments about the relative valuelessness of such common symptoms as headache, nausea, diarrhoea, and the like— when manifested by the sick patient—are equally appli-

[20]In James Tyler Kent, *Repertory of the Homoeopathic Materia Medica*, First Indian Edition, Calcutta: Hahnemann Publishing Co. Private Ltd., 1961.

cable to these symptoms when manifested in the provings of remedies. Nearly every proving will yield a group of these common symptoms, and for that reason they are of little value for treatment. What is significant are the "modalities": which conditions relieve the headache or the nausea, which aggravate them, etc. It is found that remedies can be distinguished from one another on the basis of the modalities and that these are often the key to correct prescribing.

The remedy prescribed according to the Law of Similars is "specific" to a particular disease syndrome, a particular conglomeration of symptoms, and homoeopathy thus provides an answer to the time-honored dispute in medical history over the meaning of the "specific medicine." In the orthodox tradition the "specific" has meant the medicine which was of use in a particular disease even though no explanation of its action was forthcoming, the best examples being quinine (*Cinchona*) in malaria (intermittent fever) and mercurial compounds in syphilis. Hahnemann's provings of these two substances revealed them to be homoeopathic to certain instances of their respective "diseases," and he rightly observed that their popularity over the centuries stemmed from the fact that they were truly curative in these cases because homoeopathic to their symptoms. In the light of the homoeopathic experience, therefore, "specific" means homoeopathic to a particular set of symptoms. Every medicine or substance used as a medicine is the specific remedy for the group of symptoms which it develops when proved on healthy persons. Quinine is specific to certain cases of malaria, and mercury is specific to certain syphilis syndromes. Neither is specific to all cases of disease lumped by some physicians under the headings, "malaria", or "syphilis". The specificity is not to the disease name but to certain symptom-syndromes which, in the case of malaria and syphilis, happen to be syndromes often encountered in persons suffering from these diseases.

In the orthodox tradition, on the other hand, where medicines are grouped together in terms of their general effect on some organ or system of the body, there is no method for making precise distinctions among them. The homoeopathic physician is trained to spot the one medicine, or the group of complementary medicines, out of the 2000-odd substances in the homoeopathic pharmacopoeia, which the patient before him needs. He will make regular use of perhaps 800 different medicines in his day-to-day practice. The orthodox physician today, on the contrary, lacks a method for distinguishing minutely among the many thousands of medicines on the market and will be found to make regular use of not more. than 30 to 40 medicines in his day-to-day practice, applying them in a more indiscriminate way than the homoeopathic physician.

This ability to make small distinctions among patients and among superficially similar disease processes is the natural corollary of the concern for the whole man which is central to homoeopathy. The homoeopathic physiological assumptions imply the conviction that the organism must be viewed as an integrated whole, and the Law of Similars gives the physician a technique for distinguishing the whole state of one patient from the whole state of another. Thus homoeopathy is holistic (i.e., synthesizing), as contrasted with the analytical approach of orthodox medicine. The latter bases treatment on what appear to be the common elements in a series of slightly different cases. Homoeopathy largely ignores these common elements, the prominent symptoms, and bases treatment on the small differences between one patient and another. The holism of homoeopathy applies to the medicine as well as to the patient. The provings, in principle, yield

32

all the symptoms of the remedy, and the indicated remedy is the one whose symptoms match *all* the symptoms of the patient.

Another important difference between the homoeopathic and the allopathic approaches to therapeutics stems from the homoeopathic awareness of the existence of "primary" and "secondary" symptoms of drugs. Hahnemann discovered in 1796 that any drug administered to a healthy person gives rise to two consecutive sets of symptoms, the second set being in a sense the "opposite" of the first. Hahnemann wrote, with respect to the primary and secondary symptoms of *Opium*: "A fearless elevation of spirit, a sensation of strength and high courage, an imaginative gaity, are part of the direct primary action of a moderate dose on the system: But after the lapse of eight or twelve hours an opposite state sets in, the indirect secondary action; there ensue relaxation, dejection, diffidence, peevishness, loss of memory, discomfort, fear . . ."[21] Initially he felt that both sets of symptoms were symptoms of the drug, but he later concluded that the *"secondary" symptoms expressed the reaction of the organism to the drug.* Thus it seems that the primary symptoms represent the actual effect of the drug on the organism, and the "secondary" symptoms represent the vital reaction of the organism to the drug.

The "secondary" symptoms are merely another manifestation of the reactive power of the vital force and of its ability to overcome morbific stimuli impinging upon the body from the external environment.

Hahnemann and his followers have held that the primary symptoms are the ones to be recorded in the provings. When the medicine is given whose primary symptoms are identical with the symptoms of the disease,

[21]Hahnemann, *Lesser Writings*, pp. 266–267.

the organism's reaction to the drug (expressed in the form of the secondary symptoms) will be the "opposite" of the disease symptoms and will thus neutralize or annihilate the "disorder of the vital force" which is the disease.

Hence the frequently observed "aggravation" of the disease after administration of the indicated remedy. Since the primary symptoms of the remedy are identical with the symptoms of the disease, these latter are at first intensified; this, in turn, stimulates the reactive power of the organism (the "secondary symptoms" of the provings) which overcomes and nullifies the primary symptoms (the "disease" symptoms), thus removing the disease.

2.) *The Minimum Dose.* Hahnemann's second rule was the result of his experience with the phenomenon of disease aggravation. Finding that the administration of medicines in substantial doses according to the Law of Similars led to aggravation of the patient's symptoms, he reduced his doses drastically. In the process he found that the strength of the "primary" symptoms was lessened while that of the "secondary" symptoms remained unimpaired. Since the curative effect of the remedy is a function of the "secondary" symptoms, this discovery permitted a continuing reduction in dose size.

As early as 1800 Hahnemann referred in a writing to a dose of arsenic "one ten-millionth the usual size," and after this time he made general (although not exclusive) use of the so-called ultra-molecular dose.

Since this ultra-molecular dose has become the hallmark of homoeopathy, some explanation of it must be made. Medicines are prepared for homoeopathic use by diluting one part of the original substance (if a solid) or tincture (if a liquid) in nine parts of milk sugar or of an 87% solution of alcohol and distilled water. The mixture is triturated in a mortar or succussed in a bottle for some time until the medicinal substance is uniformly distributed throughout the diluent, and it is then known as the 1 X dilution. The mixture can also be made in the proportion 1 to 99 and is then known as the 1 C dilution.

The process can be repeated as many times as is desired, and the remedies are prepared and used in all dilutions from 1 X or 1 C up to 30 X, 200 X, and beyond, the former being known as "low" and the latter as "high" dilutions.

According to the Avogadro Law, however, the number of molecules in one gram/mole of any substance is approximately 1×10^{24}. Therefore, when medicines are diluted beyond the 12 C or 24 X levels, it is statistically improbable that a single molecule of the original medicinal substance will remain in the milk-sugar or alcohol used as the diluent (assuming that a homogeneous solution has been achieved at each stage). And since homoeopathy makes frequent use of medicines diluted well beyond the Avogadro limit, these physicians are often accused of employing pure placebos.

A more controversial aspect of the dilution of remedies is the belief that the succussion and trituration of these remedies at the various stages of their preparation actually increase the power of the remedy, so that the "high dilutions" provoke a more powerful response, by the organism, than the "low dilutions."

A corollary is that some substances which are quite inert in their natural state—such as certain metals, silica, charcoal, and others—develop medicinal powers when prepared according to the above procedures. Hahnemann, for example, recommends dilutions of metallic gold as the antidote for suicidal tendencies.[22] It is felt that most mineral remedies, and those derived from the animal kingdom, act more powerfully in the higher dilutions.

[22]Hahnemann, *Lesser Writings*, p. 695.

Several comments may be made on the homoeopathic dilutions. In the first place, their value has been proven by much clinical experience. Thousands of homoeopaths have used them and are using them today. These dilutions have been found highly effective when used according to the correct indications. In the second place, a series of biological, chemical, and physical experiments have uniformly demonstrated the existence of some physico-chemical, or other, force in the ultra-molecular dilutions. In 1928, H. Junker added various substances, in dilutions up to 10^{-27}, to bacterial cultures and found that they affected the growth of the bacteria. J. Patterson and W. Boyd in Scotland found that the Schick test for diptheria was changed from positive to negative by oral administration of alum-precipitated toxoid in a dilution of 10^{-60} or of *Diphtherinum* (a homoeopathic preparation of throat swabs from diphtheria patients) in a dilution of 10^{-402}. W. Persson in Leningrad investigated the effects of dilutions up to 10^{-120} on the rate of fermentation of starch by ptyalin and on the lysis of fibrin by pepsin and trypsin; in 1954 W. Boyd announced positive results from a retest of Persson's findings with respect to the effect of dilutions of mercuric chloride up to 10^{-61} on the rate of hydrolysis of starch by diastase.[23] These findings appear to be strong evidence against any suggestion that the homoeopathic infinitesimal doses are mere placebos.[24]

Furthermore, it is worth noting that orthodox medicine has never made an effort to test this aspect of homoeopathy under controlled conditions. Criticism of the ultra-

[23]See James Stephenson, M.D., "A Review of Investigations into the Action of Substances in Dilutions Greater than 1 x 10^{-24} (Microdilutions)," *Journal of the American Institute of Homoeopathy* XLVIII (1955), 327–355.

[24]Some results of research on the physical basis of the action of microdilutions are reported in James Stephenson, M.D. and G. P. Barnard, "Fresh Evidence for a Biophysical Field," *Journal of the American Institute of Homoeopathy* LXII (1969), 73–85.

molecular dose has been strictly *a priori*—with vague references to common sense which is a notoriously unreliable guide in medical matters.

Use of the ultra-molecular dose, in any case, is not an essential principle of homoeopathy. Hahnemann insisted on the "minimum dose", which is an ambiguous concept in view of the associated doctrine that increased dilution of the substance actually enhances its power. Homoeopathic physicians, like Hahnemann himself, make use of the whole range of dilutions, from the lowest to the highest.

3.) *The Single Remedy*. Hahnemann's third rule requires the physician to administer one remedy at a time. Here again his rule contrasts with orthodox practice which permits the use of several drugs at once or in combination.

The homoeopathic principle is not arbitrary but stems logically from the other elements of the homoeopathic system. The physician may give only one drug at a time because the provings are only of a single substance. The physician may not give two remedies at once (i.e., on the ground that their combined symptoms match all of the symptoms of the patient) because, when two remedies are administered at the same time, they yield additional symptoms which are neither those of substance A nor of substance B, but of A and B combined. Administration of two remedies at the same time introduces an unknown into the picture, and the purpose of Hahnemann's new method was to eliminate just such speculative and unreliable procedures from medicine.

Homoeopathy is in no way averse to the use of chemical compounds *provided they have been proved as such.* Thus, *Ferrum metallicum* yields one set of symptoms, and *Phosphorus* yields another set. Phosphate of iron (*Ferrum phosphoricum*) yields symptoms of both *Ferrum metallicum* and *Phosphorus*, but, in addition, has a distinctive action not found in either of its components. The characteristic symptoms produced by *Ferrum phosphoricum* mark it as a distinctive single remedy, and it must be prescribed on the basis of the symptoms from its own proving, not on the basis of a mixture of *Ferrum metallicum* and *Phosphorus* symptoms.

The homoeopathic materia medica contains provings of numerous such chemical compounds: potassium sulphate, protoiodide of mercury, sodium carbonate, to mention only a few.

In orthodox practice, the use of medicinal mixtures is justified on the ground that each medicine has a specific function inside the body and is directed "against" some specific aspect of the disease in question. Homoeopaths disapprove of this practice not only because the medicines are not given in accordance with the Law of Similars, but also because such mixtures yield new and unpredictable combined effects which may be harmful to the patient. Here, as elsewhere, the homoeopathic approach is consistently holistic—demanding the matching of the whole symptomatology of the patient with the symptomatology of a single remedy.

4.) *The Theory of Chronic Diseases.* A final aspect of the homoeopathic system is Hahnemann's theory of chronic diseases. After practicing his new system for nearly two decades, Hahnemann found that in many cases the symptoms of acute diseases disappeared only temporarily and subsequently either recurred or were replaced by a new pattern of symptoms. The patient was not permanently cured, and his health was not permanently improved. This led him to the conclusion that underlying these acute diseases were a number of chronic "miasms" or chronic diseases which had to be cured first—before a lasting cure of the supervening acute disease could be effected.

In 1828 he published a work which hypothesized the existence of three basic chronic diseases; psora, syphilis, and sycosis (gonorrhoea). These three chronic diseases, which assume the most protean forms (Hahnemann wrote five volumes of their symptoms), were to be cured by *Sulphur, Mercurius,* and *Thuja (Arbor vitae)* respectively.

Hahnemann's theory of chronic diseases is a departure from his principle of the uniqueness of each individual case and a step in the direction of reliance on the disease entity. For this and other reasons it provoked fierce controversy in homoeopathic ranks which lasted for decades. Today, however, a consensus has been reached on this point, which can be summarized as follows.

While it is felt that Hahnemann's symptomatic description of these three chronic diseases, and the remedies he selected for them, are correct, there is less agreement on the causal relationship between these miasms and their respective acute forms, that is, the acute forms of psora (the "itch"), syphilis, and gonorrhoea.[25] Therefore, at the present time, Hahnemann's chronic-disease theory has been converted into a principle of homoeopathic practice. When the indicated remedy fails to cure, or effects a cure which is not permanent, one of the chronic-disease remedies is probably indicated, and when this remedy has run its course, the indicated remedies for the acute disease are seen to be once again effective. Thus, a contemporary homoeopathic materia medica states, with respect to sulphur: "When carefully selected remedies fail to act, especially in acute diseases, it frequently arouses the reactionary powers of the organism . . . prescribed for complaints that relapse."[26]

[25]Dhawale, *Principles and Practice of Homoeopathy,* Volume I, Bombay, 1967, pp. 443 ff.

[26]W. Boericke, *Materia Medica With Repertory,* Ninth Edition, Philadelphia, 1927, p. 520.

In conclusion, it should be stressed that the rationale for prescribing the remedy in homoeopathic practice is very different from its rationale in orthodox practice. The homoeopath views disease as a derangement or disturbance of the body's economy, of the vital force. Since this disturbance cannot be known directly by the physician, because of the complexity of the internal processes involved, it must be cognized indirectly by means of the patient's symptoms. The symptoms reveal the course taken by the vital force in counteracting the morbific environmental stimulus. The remedy is administered with the aim of helping the organism to react along these lines. The only remedy which can produce this effect is the *single substance*, administered in the *minimum dose*, and in *strict conformity with the Law of Similars*.

Thus, the homoeopathic refusal to base remedy selection on bacteriological factors has a logical basis. While no homoeopath denies the indisputable fact that germs, bacteria, viruses, etc., can cause or aggravate diseases in various ways,[27] this does not mean that the most appropriate mode of therapy is one which attempts to "kill" the germ or bacterium or virus within the organism. Germs are merely another type of morbific external force. Once inside the body, they promote a reaction just like any other such stimulus. In bacterial diseases, as in all others, the homoeopath attempts to further the reaction of the organism, and experience shows well that this procedure is as successful in this class of diseases as in others.

Thus, the homoeopath disapproves of the use of bactericidal medicines, feeling that killing the assumed bacterial or viral disease "cause" within the body does not lead to a

[27]In 1832, Hahnemann suggested that the cause of the Asiatic cholera epidemic of that year was probably "an enormous . . . brood of excessively minute, invisible, living creatures" (*Lesser Writings*, p. 758). He still called for remedies prescribed on a symptomatic basis. Many of these remedies were taken over by allopathic medicine.

true or permanent cure, since it in no way strengthens the organism. In fact, this type of medication may well weaken the organism and affect adversely its inherent recuperative powers, leaving the patient prone to a relapse or to infection with another disease. It is well-known that antibiotics can at times upset the balance of microorganisms within the body and thus permit the ingress of pathogenic varieties.

Similarly, in the homoeopathic view, the other typical medicines used in orthodox practice—substances which stimulate or depress some physiological function, deal only with particular manifestations of the disease process and fail to reach the root.

Killing the germ inside the body does not eliminate the disease cause. The "cause" is not the germ but the pre-existing state of the organism which permits the germ to exist and multiply there. Enhancing or blocking some physiological function does not remove the disease cause but only diverts the vital force into different channels. The "cause" is the preexisting state of the organism which in time gives rise to an observable pathological process. It is non-material and cannot be cognized directly. Knowledge of it is obtained only through the minute homoeopathic analysis of the patient's symptoms. This cause can be removed only through administration of the similar remedy.

It is even possible that the antibacterial and antiviral medicines, metabolic inhibitors, and other medicines commonly employed in today's allopathic practice actually predispose the patient to such degenerative diseases as arthritis, heart trouble, and cancer. The increasing frequency of these complaints, in the homoeopathic view, is partly the consequence of the use of powerful allopathic remedies which affect the body in an incorrect and ultimately harmful way.

IV. THE PLACE OF PATHOLOGICAL DIAGNOSIS IN HOMOEOPATHY

We have been stressing the homoeopathic rejection of pathological diagnosis as a guide to selection of the remedy, but that does not mean that the modern homoeopathic physician denies any value to pathology. Here we will attempt to clarify the much controverted issue of the relationship between pathology and homoeopathic practice.

In the first place, the homoeopathic physician does refuse to base his prescription of the remedy, *in diseases which are curable through the use of drugs*, on pathological diagnosis. The progress from symptoms to pathological entity to the curative medicine is an allopathic procedure which is not employed in homoeopathy and whose value is denied by the homoeopathic physician. His method moves from the totality of the symptoms directly to the remedy, largely bypassing the pathological stage with its uncertainties.

Over the years this procedure has given rise to much criticism from orthodox practitioners who state that homoeopathic treatment is "symptomatic"—i.e., not directed against the "disease" but only against the symptoms.

A careful analysis of this argument, however, reveals it to be merely a remnant of the disease-entity way of thinking. It reflects the belief that the "disease itself" is somehow in existence within, and independent of, the body. The presence of this entity is thought to produce certain symptoms, and the "mere" removal of these symptoms is not viewed as equivalent to curing the "disease."

Homoeopathy, however, regards disease as a distortion, disharmony, or misdirection of the body's vital force. If a medicine is administered which covers the *totality* of the patient's symptoms and thus removes *all* of these symptoms—so that the patient feels entirely well afterwards and appears in excellent health, who is to say that the "disease" has not been removed, that the patient has not been cured?

Hahnemann answered this criticism in the following words: "It is not conceivable nor can it be proved by any experience in the world, that, after removal of all the symptoms of the disease, and the entire collection of the perceptible phenomena, there should or could remain anything else besides health, or that the morbid alteration in the interior could remain unaltered."[28] "In the cure effected by the removal of the whole of the perceptible signs and symptoms of the disease, the internal alteration of the vital principle to which the disease is due—consequently the whole of the disease—is at the same time removed."[29] As a later commentator has put it, "*Cessat effectus, cessat causa.*"[30]

Of fundamental importance to Hahnemann's dictum is the idea that the *totality* of the symptoms must be re-

[28] Hahnemann, *Organon*, Section 8.

[29] *Ibid.*, Section 17.

[30] *Ibid.*, Introduction by James Krauss, M.D. ("When the effect ceases, so does the cause").

moved by the *single remedy*.[31] The idea that the symptomatology of the disease must match that of the remedy *to the last detail* is a far cry from what is called symptomatic prescribing in orthodox practice, where several different medicines are administered because of their presumed action "against" several of the patient's symptoms.

The next problem is the role of pathology in the total management of the patient. It must be admitted that this question has not always been properly understood in the past by the homoeopaths themselves, as they have often confused the purely pharmaceutical side of medicine with the whole of medical practice. A more balanced view prevails at present, however, and it can be summarized as follows:

1) Pathological knowledge has the important function of demarcating the cases which are, in principle, amenable to drug treatment from those where some other type of treatment, such as surgery, dietary adjustment, or manipulative therapy, may be indicated. Diseases caused by defective diet are best treated by improving the diet, and it may be found that no medicine at all is needed thereafter. Deficiency diseases can often be spotted by symptoms alone, but in many cases pathological investigations are also needed. The same is true for diseases requiring surgery. While homoeopaths have always held that surgery is less used in homoeopathic practice than in orthodox practice, there is no theoretical objection to it. Often its necessity is revealed through pathological investigations, and it may be employed whenever needed. Homoeopathy, furthermore, is fully compatible with the

---

[31]*Ibid.*, Section 70. It is understood that the development of the disease will usually require different remedies—matching the changing symptom-pattern. But two medicines are never to be given *simultaneously*.

various forms of manipulative therapy, and homoeopaths, more than other physicians, have recognized the value of these types of treatment.

2) Just as pathological knowledge helps to demarcate the diseases curable by drug therapy from those which are not, it also helps to distinguish the symptoms of the patient's altered vital force from those symptoms which may be the secondary consequences of some gross pathological alteration. An authority notes: *"frequency of micturition*, with a morbid growth impacted in the pelvis, would not help you in the choice of a remedy. It would be a symptom secondary to gross pathological change; not a symptom expressing the patient herself, but a symptom merely dependent on mechanical pressure; promptly relieved by the removal of the tumor."[32]

3) Another important use of pathological knowledge is in demarcating cases with favorable prognosis from those in which the prognosis is unfavorable. When the pathological changes are far advanced, and the vital organs have been seriously affected, use of a powerful and deepacting homoeopathic remedy may so disturb the economy as to lead to death. The homoeopathic literature contains a number of instances of this. Thus, when the prognosis is unfavorable, the homoeopath is often best advised to employ superficial and palliative remedies which do not attempt to provoke a far-reaching restorative process, since the patient's recuperative powers may not be equal to the task of cure. This state of the organism is often to be discovered through use of the common diagnostic procedures.

4) A final use of pathology, mentioned in one of the leading contemporary homoeopathic texts, is the follow-

---

[32]J. T. Kent, *Repertory of the Homoeopathy Materia Medica*, Introduction by Margaret Tyler, M.D., p. viii.

ing: When treating such epidemic diseases as typhoid or cholera, in which the same group of homoeopathic remedies is usually indicated, the physician may benefit from a knowledge of the pathological changes which indicate the particular epidemic process. Then the correct remedy can be administered at an early stage when the symptomatology is still diffuse and unclear, i.e., before the typical symptoms characterizing the particular epidemic process have had time to develop.

This latter procedure is still, in principle, identical with prescribing on a symptomatic basis. The pathological indications enable the physician to resolve which of the patient's unclear symptoms are of significance for prescribing.

Practitioners are agreed, however, that this procedure carries a serious risk of abuse, for its apparent short-cutting of the laborious stage of symptom analysis. The general rule remains, as always, that remedies are to be selected on the basis of the symptoms.

Pathological knowledge is imprecise. It does not permit of individualization. That is why it is rejected as a guide to remedy selection. A modern authority has written:

> "Supposing many drugs *had* been pushed so far as to produce Pneumonia, for instance, each would produce not only a Pneumonia with symptoms peculiar to itself, but would also elicit symptoms peculiar to individual provers, so that you would still need to individualize, in order to cure. Pathologists know that drugs produce Pneumonia or Sciatica; what they do not know is that they produce a *modified* Sciatica or Pneumonia."[33]

Furthermore, there is no way in which this could be changed. While remedies could, in principle, be proved for

[33] J. T. Kent, *Repertory of the Homoeopathic Materia Medica*, Introduction by Margaret Tyler, M.D., p. viii.

pathological indications, this would be extremely laborious, and a thorough pathological picture of the remedy's effect would demand an autopsy of the prover! And what would be the point? The symptoms already provide more subtle and differentiated pictures of drug effects than could ever be obtained from pathological investigations.

V. THE SEARCH FOR A SCIENTIFIC THERAPEUTICS

The fundamental problem of medicine is how to establish therapeutics on a scientific basis. The argument between the homoeopaths and the orthodox physicians is, *inter alia*, a dispute over the meaning of scientific method in therapeutics. At present, both groups of physicians claim their method to be scientific. Since the methods are in many respects opposed to one another, they clearly cannot both be scientific. Our problem now is to ascertain whether homoeopathy or orthodox medicine is more entitled to claim the honor of being a "scientific" form of therapeutics.

1.) *The Role of "Art" in Medical Practice.* A preliminary issue is the proper importance of the "artistic" component of medicine. Physicians are fond of insisting that therapeutics must always be ultimately an "artistic" endeavor. Disease parameters are too indefinite and changeable, and there are too many imponderabilia, it is said, for precise and rigid scientific standards to apply.

We sympathize with this view to the extent that it is not designed to cover up incompetence. Too often the claim for artistic freedom is merely a claim for maximum latitude in medical practice. But such freedom, while gratifying to the practitioner, always entails a risk to the patient. While we admit that therapeutics contains an "artistic" dimension, we also feel that its magnitude should be diminished to the utmost.

Art should be a supplement to scientific knowledge, not a substitute for it. It would be odd if engineers were to pontificate about the role of art in bridge-building, as if this were to take the place of the requisite knowledge of strength of materials. Engineers are inhibited from so doing because, in their profession, when art encroaches too much on science, the bridges fall down.

Unfortunately, the same is not so clearly true for medicine. Patients may live despite their physician's best efforts or die because of them, but the cause-and-effect relationship is more obscure when the workman's materials are not steel and concrete but the living, vital, reactive human organism.

In any case, the existence of an artistic dimension in therapeutics should not preclude us from attempting a rational analysis of the principles and procedures which might make this discipline scientific.

2.) *The Modern Allopathic Definition of "Scientific Medicine"*. Discussion of this issue is complicated, as is any discussion of medical questions, by the general confusion over terms and definitions and by the lack of agreement on the meaning of "scientific method" in medicine.

Spokesmen for orthodox medicine will generally claim that their procedures are scientific to the extent that they embody precise measurements. Thus the various diagnostic and other tests employed, which are based upon recognized chemical and physical principles, are supposed to be scientific and to make the practice of medicine scientific. But the unreliability and ambiguity of diagnostic procedures are well-known and admitted on all sides, and these procedures could thus not be "scientific" in any ordinary sense of the word. At this point the physician usually falls back upon the concept of the physician's "tact" or artistic sense: "Judgment is the essence of the clinical method in its fullness,"[34] diagnosis is "the product not of guessing but of a sifted experience by which the significant is recognized with such rapidity that the steps of reasoning are not discernible to the uninitiated."[35]

If diagnosis is not a scientific procedure, the next step—the selection of treatment—can hardly be scientific either. Allopathic diagnosis never points unambiguously to a single medicine; there is no necessary or immediate relationship between the diagnosis and the remedy. The physician's judgment is always called into play.

Confronted with these arguments the orthodox physician will respond that while medicine is not scientific with respect to any individual case, it compensates for this by proceeding on the basis of the statistical averages of cases. Statistical techniques are supposed to be especially valuable in providing evidence of the efficacy of drugs.

Both approaches to establishing medicine on a scientific basis are thus premised upon acceptance of the concept of the disease entity. In the first case, accurate measurement of the disease parameters is supposed to be sufficient to determine whether or not a particular patient is suffering from a particular "disease". In the second case, the statistical procedure can be valid only if all the patients investigated are indeed suffering from the same "disease".

[34]Sir James Spence, "The Methodology of Clinical Science", *The Lancet*, September 26, 1953, p. 629.

[35]F. M. R. Walshe, "On Clinical Medicine", *The Lancet*, December 16, 1950, p. 784.

The disease entity plays as pivotal a role in today's orthodox therapeutics as it did for Galen. This concept was refined with Pierre Louis' introduction of statistics into medicine in the early nineteenth century and immediately encountered the most serious methodological and philosophical objections. The essence of these objections has always been that finding a statistical mean or average between unlike things does not make them like. An average could be found between six oranges and six apples, but it would have no physical meaning; nothing corresponds to it in the physical world, especially in a field such as medicine where the ultimate reality is always a single individual person. These ideas have been presented in their most trenchant form by Claude Bernard:

> Another very frequent application of mathematics to biology is the use of averages which, in medicine and physiology, leads, so to speak, necessarily, to error. There are doubtless several reasons for this: But the greatest obstacle to applying calculation to physiological phenomena is still, at bottom, the excessive complexity which prevents their being definite and comparable one with another. By destroying the biological character of phenomena, the use of *averages* in physiology and medicine usually gives only apparent accuracy to the results . . . Aside from physical and chemical, there are physiological averages, or what we might call average descriptions of phenomena, which are even more false. Let me assume that a physician collects a great many individual observations of a disease and that he makes an average description of symptoms observed in the individual cases; he will thus have a description that will never be matched in nature. So in physiology we must never make average descriptions of experiments, because the true relations of phenomena disappear in the average . . . averages must therefore be rejected, because they confuse, while aiming to unify, and distort, while aiming to simplify . . .[36]

[36]Claude Bernard, *An Introduction to the Study of Experimental Medicine*, New York: Dover, 1957, pp. 134–135.

52

It is odd indeed that the great French physiologist, who is usually cited as the foremost philosopher of contemporary orthodox therapeutic method, should in fact have rejected the fundamental concept upon which this method is founded. But the nineteenth-century controversy over the use of statistics in medicine is presumed to have been settled, and Claude Bernard's spiritual descendants have until recently been content to leave it so.

Interest in the significance of the statistical average for medicine was reawakened with the 1962 Kefauver-Harris amendments to the Food, Drug, and Cosmetic Act. The 1962 law for the first time compelled drug manufacturers to develop statistical evidence for the effectiveness of the medicines which they wanted to produce and sell. Prior to this time the clinical testing of medicines had been fairly haphazard; afterwards it became a large-scale affair and has been discussed much more comprehensively in the medical literature.

The upshot has been a new attack on the disease-entity concept. The theoretically simple procedure of gathering together a group of people with the "same" disease and evaluating their response to a drug has been found to encounter unexpected obstacles. Ensuring "group homogeneity" or "group comparability" turns out to be far more difficult than had been supposed. A professional medical statistician comments:

> One of the basic limitations under which clinical research often has to be performed is the relatively small number of patients available for a given study, particularly with respect to the large number of variables which may, at least in theory, affect behavior or symptomatology . . . It is . . . quite difficult to obtain strictly comparable groups of patients for use in an extensive model. Manifest or hidden differences in patient

53

characteristics, in view of the necessarily small sample sizes, can play havoc with significance levels in either direction.[37]

The problem is especially acute in the chemotherapy of mental diseases:

Most psychiatric syndromes have neither generally accepted causes (etiologies) nor treatments whose efficacy is unchallenged. Consequently, patients used in drug trials can only be defined by diagnostic categories or by the presence or absence of particular signs and symptoms. For example, doctors in one hospital may diagnose as schizophrenic only those patients who have been in the hospital two or more years. Other doctors in hospital might consider that some of the patients should have been diagnosed differently, e.g., as having depressions, psychopathic personalities, and even brain damage and epilepsy. If the sample of schizophrenia patients being studied consists of those who have been ill under one year, the discrepancies in diagnosis will be even greater.[38]

Sometimes the difficulty is expressed in terms of "defining the disease" or "defining the pathological process":

We can cite other kinds of sampling problems which can confuse the investigator. There is, for example, evidence that therapeutic trials on the management of atypical pneumonia have disagreed in their conclusions at least partly because of difficulties in defining the disease. It now appears fairly definite that the Eaton agent, when it is involved in causing primary atypical pneumonia, is quite susceptible to broad-spectrum antibiotics. It seems likely that other varieties of atypical pneumonia caused by true viruses do not respond to such antibiotics. It has been pointed out that rheumatic fever covers a broad spectrum of disease, and that one can affect the results of a therapeutic trial dramatically by failing to take into account factors known

[37]J. B. Chassan, "Statistical Inference and the Single Case in Clinical Design", *Psychiatry*, XXIII (1960), pp. 173, 184.

[38]A. Hoffer and H. Osmond, "Double-Blind Clinical Trials", *Journal of Neuropsychiatry*,, II (1960–1961), p. 222.

to affect prognosis in this disease . . . Coronary artery disease and cancer are other miscellaneous labels for a variety of ills, and it behooves us . . . to be circumspect in our classification of disease, so that we may sharpen the precision of our results and the ability to extrapolate from them.[39]

Problems are encountered also in the second stage of the experiment—evaluation of the patient's response to the drug. The biological effect of a drug can never be determined *a priori* from a theoretical analysis of its molecular structure.[40] Hence, one primordial assumption of the allopathic method in therapeutics—that the mechanism of action of the medicine can be known—is thus far unproven.

Consequently, the allopathic physician must attempt to measure the drug effect empirically and generalize these results over the whole patient population. But this gives rise to the same procedural difficulty as in the case of diagnosis, for patients react very differently to the same drug. The modern literature emphasizes that drug effects "are never identical in all patients or even in a given patient on different occasions."[41] "An occasional individual responds to a drug in a fashion qualitatively different from the usual response . . . Such a response is called 'idiosyncrasy' . . . "[42]

The patient's personality and emotional state have a considerable influence on his sensitivity to the medication (mental and emotional symptoms are, of course, very important for homoeopathic prescribing):

[39]Louis Lasagna in Paul Talalay, ed., *Drugs in Our Society*, Baltimore: Johns Hopkins, 1964, p. 100.

[40]See notes 11, 12, and 13, above.

[41]L. S. Goodman and Alfred Gilman, *The Pharmacological Basis of Therapeutics*, Third Edition, New York: Macmillan and Co., 1965, p. 21.

[42]Victor A. Drill, *Pharmacology in Medicine*, p. 1/19.

The emotional state of the individual is crucial in evaluation of nitrites. Patients with angina pectoris, not all of them, but many of them, tend to be somewhat dependent upon their physician as a bulwark between them and the sudden death that they fear. The placebo effect is strong in suggestible individuals with angina pectoris, and relief of angina may be effected by a reduction in anxiety due to the personality of the physician rather than to the nitrites administered.[43]

In much the same way that some species of laboratory animals are superior to others for particular experiments in the laboratory, the choice of a suitable subject is often a critical matter for an investigation in man. Thus, while the best subject will tend to make the method more sensitive, unsuitable subjects may dilute the response to drugs and make the method so insensitive that it is unable to detect the particular drug reaction under investigation and, therefore, regardless of the activity of the drug or effectiveness of the controls, provides only a negative answer . . . In studies involving subjective criteria, excessively phlegmatic subjects tend to desensitize the method by failure to react with normal sensitivity while exceedingly neurotic and overreactive or highly suggestible patients tend to compromise the sensitivity of the method through wide swings of mood and attitude as the result both of placebo and of active medication. In general, unusual and abnormal, as well as hypersensitive and resistant subjects desensitize evaluations.[44]

All of this criticism stems from the elementary proposition first voiced by Claude Bernard, that *unlike things cannot be made like by any amount of statistical manipulation.* The British geneticist, Lancelot Hogben, has pointed out:

It is not enough to show that drug A is better than drug B on the average. One is invited to ask, 'For which people (and why)

[43] *Proceedings of the Institute on Drug Literature Evaluation, Philadelphia, Pennsylvania, March 11–15, 1968.* Washington, D.C., 1968, p. 95.

[44] Walter Modell, "The Sensitivity and Validity of Drug Evaluations in Man," *Clinical Pharmacology and Therapeutics,* I (1960), p. 769.

is drug A better than drug B and vice-versa? If drug A cures 40% and drug B cures 60%, perhaps the right choice of drug for each person would result in 100% cures'.[45]

That much of the criticism is finding its mark can be seen from the emotional reaction of Louis Lasagna, who writes:

> We are, to be sure, all different from one another, and it is probably true that one could listen to hundreds of lungs during the pneumonia season and not find two that sounded exactly alike. But this is not the same as saying that there are no common features in such patients or that therapeutically one starts from scratch every time one faces a patient with pneumonia. If this were so, medical teaching would be impossible, and the practice of medicine chaos, or at least anarchy. The problem of individual differences is indeed a challenging one . . . but it is no reason for paralytic despair.[46]

The author's use of such hyperbolic expressions as "paralytic despair", "chaos", and "anarchy" reflect an unconscious concern lest the whole method break down—lest someone come forward and point out that the emperor does not have any clothes on after all.

And the concern is entirely justified, as all contemporary discussion of therapeutic method in the orthodox school emphasizes the weaknesses, both theoretical and practical, of the disease-entity concept. And if this cornerstone of the allopathic therapeutic edifice does indeed rest on sand, the whole structure must be shaky.

Let us examine allopathic therapeutic method from a more theoretical angle. What is called "scientific method" is only a technique for testing hypotheses against the facts of experience. The application of scientific method to

[45]Paraphrased in *Annual Review of Medicine* IX (1958), p. 349.
[46]In Paul Talalay, ed., *Drugs in Our Society*, pp. 93–94.

therapeutics would be as follows: It would be hypothesized, on whatever grounds seem sufficient, that disease X is cured or alleviated by medicine Y. Whatever scientific input lies behind it, the outcome is a proposition in the above form. The physician's task is to verify the truth of this proposition.

This is done by translating the hypothesis into facts or data which are commensurable with the data of medical experience. At this crucial point, however, allopathic procedure is defective, since its hypothesis can only take the form: "Persons suffering from *disease entity* X are cured by medicine Y." But, as we have seen, there exists no precise relationship between the hypothesized disease entity and the ultimate facts of experience—the sick patients. The results anticipated from application of the hypothesis cannot be defined in terms of the physician's day-to-day reality, the patients who come into his office, but only in terms of an abstraction. The individual case cannot be adequately described in itself but has meaning only as the representative of some hypothetical entity.

The result is that one hypothesis can be verified only in terms of another hypothesis. Proof of the hypothesis that "Disease X is cured by medicine Y" is dependent upon the further hypothesis that "Such-and-such patient-population manifesting such-and-such symptoms and pathology form disease entity X." The circularity of the reasoning is complete when it is realized that the second hypothesis is sometimes demonstrated in terms of the first: The fact that such-and-such a patient is suffering from disease X is proved by the effectiveness of medicine Y in treating this patient.

Whatever the above procedures may be, they are not scientific. Orthodox medicine has no way of testing its hypotheses against unambiguous sensory data. The disease entity is a statistical mean or average of a number of different cases, and its description may not match the description of a single one of the observed cases. The outcome is a methodological morass in which one defective hypothesis is temporarily propped up by others equally defective, and it is hardly surprising that orthodox pathological and therapeutic theory pass through the bewildering changes and gyrations which are apparent to any student of medical history.

Defenders of modern allopathic therapeutics often maintain that it must be accepted despite its methodological defects because there is no alternative. However, homoeopathy does offer an alternative which eliminates the principal methodological insufficiencies noted above.

3) *The Homoeopathic View of "Scientific Medicine"*. Hahnemann's aim was to introduce a rational order and method into the therapeutic use of drugs. It only remains to determine whether or not this method is "scientific", i.e., meets the requirements of scientific method.

It has already been noted that homoeopathy offers a different principle for classifying diseases, namely, in terms of the medicines which cure them. It would be more correct, however, to state that homoeopathy offers a technique for distinguishing disease conditions on a symptomatic basis, since the symptoms which point to the remedy at the same time indicate to the physician the disease from which the patient is suffering. This idea is understood with difficulty by persons trained in orthodox medicine. who immediately think of homoeopathy as effecting nothing more than superficial symptomatic cures. But the homoeopathic use of symptoms differs greatly from the use of symptoms in orthodox practice; it is never one symptom, or even several symptoms, which are taken by the physician as his guide, but the whole dynamic pattern of the symptoms. No single symptom has significance by itself. Only in the context of the patient's whole syndrome—*which is at the same time the symptom-syndrome of the curative medicine*—does the individual symptom take on meaning. The patients are not shunted into speculative pathological categories but are classified in terms of the meaningful symptoms. And the symptoms which are meaningful are the ones which at the same time point to the curative medicine.[47]

Thus, the homoeopathic method has solved the problem of establishing an unambiguous definition of the primary data—the individual cases of disease, the individual patients. Each is described in the minutest way, and the proof that these descriptions are valid and accurate is that they have withstood the test of more than 150 years. What is often seen as a weakness of homoeopathy—that it is unchanged in its essentials—is actually an advantage. A well-observed symptom is an unchanging datum. Careful physicians for generations have found that the homoeopathic characterizations of disease processes are as true for them as for their predecessors. The homoeopathic system is a sturdy and stable edifice because it rests on this firm methodological foundation.

In this way homoeopathy reduces to a minimum the artistic component in medical practice. To quote James Tyler Kent:

"The records of confirmed and verified provings stand as so many recorded facts.

[47]The idea of distinguishing diseased states in terms of the medicines which cure them has recently been proposed in an allopathic medical journal. Complaining that the emphasis on disease categories has caused the production of medicines with undesirable side-effects, Drs. A. Hoffer and H. Osmond have proposed that a search be made for more specific drugs. They call for a focus on the drug and not on the disease—"the essence of this method is to find the clinical situation which will respond to a known chemical. This should not frighten clinicians, for it is one of the standard methods in medicine. . . . " (A. Hoffer and H. Osmond, "Double-Blind Clinical Trials," *Journal of Neuro-psychiatry* II (1961), p. 222).

The symptoms of the sick man are recorded as so many facts.
The similarity between the two is the only variable quantity,
and this is a matter of art; and art is always a variable
quantity."[48]

And not only are the homoeopathic descriptions of diseases and medicines precise and accurate, they are also systematic. The primordial difficulty of medicine is the welter of subtly differentiated diseased states, the huge volume of information offered to the physician, whose interpretation demands some methodological guide. These careful and precise homoeopathic disease descriptions would be of little value in the absence of a generalizing principle enabling the physician to establish some order among the masses of conflicting and contradictory symptoms and cases. Physicians of ancient and modern times have sought this pattern, this guide to practice, in the prominent symptoms, the striking pathological processes. The homoeopaths reject this approach as unreliable and scientifically invalid and propose another one which is that the myriad cases of disease be ordered in terms of the medicines which cure them, or, as we have observed above, that cases be distinguished from one another on the basis of their symptoms.

The detailed symptomatic descriptions of disease employed in homoeopathic practice are not the work of mere artistry but are a disciplined scientific approach to the problem of disease characterization because, *by virtue of the Law of Similars*, such descriptions at the same time characterize the curative medicine. The Law of Similars establishes a precise relationship between the symptoms of the disease and the symptomatology of the curative medicine. The more precise the description of the patient's symptoms, the more precise are the indications of the curative remedy.

[48]Kent, *Lesser Writings*, p. 206.

61

The next step follows naturally. Giving the patient the indicated medicine is equivalent to applying the hypothesis that *this particular case* is cured by the similar remedy. It is a scientific test of the Law of Similars, and if the patient recovers, the truth of this doctrine can be provisionally accepted. Of course, a single recovery proves nothing in particular. But when the physician has treated hundreds and thousands of patients and has found that: 1) most of them recover, 2) recovery is in accordance with Hering's Law, and 3) the recovered patients remain healthy and are comparatively free from chronic physical and mental disease later in life, he is justified in concluding that the Law of Similars is a scientific guide to medical practice.

Further support for the scientific status of homoeopathy is found in the realization that its knowledge is stable and cumulative, as opposed to allopathic medical knowledge which is unstable and non-cumulative. Carrol Dunham in 1885 defined a scientific medicine as one possessing the "capability of infinite progress in each of its elements without detriment to its integrity as a whole."[49] Homoeopathy has remained unchanged in its essentials for nearly 200 years. Its practitioners find that many of the 19th-century books are still valuable and that the experience of the forefathers is still valid. New pharmacological knowledge can be integrated into the existing framework of doctrine without this making obsolete what has gone before.

This contrasts with allopathic medicine whose disease categories shift with changes in pathological fashions. Signs and symptoms which are considered significant at one period in history lose their meaning in another period and are replaced by new and different indications.

[49]Carrol Dunham, *Homoeopathy, The Science of Therapeutics*, Philadelphia: F. E. Boericke, 1885, p. 13.

Spokesmen for allopathic medicine extol this as the veriest proof that their doctrines are scientific, but one may rightly wonder if the continued instability of fundamental pathological doctrines does not rather reflect a methodological weakness. One often overlooked consequence is the impossibility of constructing a medical doctrine which will remain stable over time. Any statistical analysis based on disease entities is invalidated when these entities disappear and are replaced by new ones.

In medicine, as in so many other areas of life, unceasing change has long been regarded as evidence of progress, but in the latter part of the twentieth century people have come to realize that change in and for itself is not an unalloyed good. The practice of medicine could only benefit if, instead of meekly accepting every supposedly world-shaking discovery destined to revolutionize the healing art, physicians sought the permanent and unchanging in the phenomena of health and disease.

VI. HOMOEOPATHY AND MODERN MEDICINE

Homoeopathic medicine flourished in the United States after 1830 and by 1900 had more than 15,000 practitioners—one-sixth of the entire medical profession. It was temporarily pushed into the background, however, in the age of Pasteur and Koch when bacteriology dominated all of medical thought. During these years every disease was thought to be of bacterial origin, and the new science seemed to promise a "magic bullet" against each germ.

Dietary aspects of treatment were neglected, as was consideration of the patient's natural resistance to disease. It was entirely forgotten that the disease germ needs a congenial environment in which to grow and that the homoeopathic method of fortifying this internal environment, of stimulating the patient's natural reactive power, was still the best approach to the therapeutics of bacterial diseases.

Since the earliest years of homoeopathy's introduction into this country the spokesmen for medical orthodoxy had opposed it. Physicians who adopted this mode of practice were expelled from their medical societies, and consultation with homoeopathic practitioners was specifically prohibited by the AMA's Code of Ethics.[50] In the early 20th century this inherent prejudice of orthodox medicine against homoeopathy seemed to be legitimized by the findings of science. The homoeopathic approach appeared to be outdated—superseded by the new activist orientation offered by bacteriology. For several decades the principles embodied in the homoeopathic system have been under a cloud.

Today, however, the pendulum is swinging back. Not only has modern medicine failed to provide the promised cures for all of man's ills but it has itself become a major source of sickness. The powerful drugs used in orthodox practice are causing a true epidemic of iatro-genic disease. As early as 1966 the American College of Physicians estimated that about 5% of hospital admissions were for drug-induced diseases, and the incidence has been rising steadily.[51] Later surveys at university hospitals have found that more than 15% of the patients had iatro-genic illnesses.[52]

The *Bulletin of the Atomic Scientists* has observed in this connection that if only 0.1% of all hospital admissions were to die of drug reactions, the deaths would approach 29,000 a year, and iatrogenic death would constitute a "major public health problem, comparable in importance to infectious disease, cancer of the breast, and nephritis as a cause of mortality."[53]

While these figures are disagreeable in themselves, they fail to take into account all possible consequences

[50]On the nineteenth-century relations between homoeopathic and orthodox physicians, see the author's 1969 doctoral dissertation at Columbia University: *Political and Social Aspects of Nineteenth-Century Medicine in the United States: The Formation of the American Medical Association and Its Struggle With the Homoeopathic and Eclectic Physicians.*

[51]*Newsweek*, May 2, 1966, p. 66.

[52]*Bulletin of the Atomic Scientists*, January, 1969, p. 11.

[53]*Loc. cit.*

of the abuse of drugs in contemporary orthodox practice. Some patients react instantaneously to improper medication, but what of the patient whose reaction takes weeks, months, or perhaps years to manifest itself? The statistics will indicate that he was "cured" of his first ailment and then fell ill a second time with some new disorder; but if the "cure" was only apparent, being a mere suppression of some of the prominent symptoms, the patient actually remained ill the whole time.

The homoeopathic theory of chronic disease suggests that this is precisely what is happening—that the rising incidence of chronic disease is, in part, the consequence of the improper use of drugs by allopathic physicians. Cancer in young children, once comparatively rare, becomes increasingly common. A recent investigation even found a connection between a medicine (diethylstilbestrol) given pregnant women and the onset of cancer, twenty years later, in their *daughters*.[54]

Cancer, arthritis, heart disease, and others are steadily increasing their toll of the nation's health, replacing the infectious disease which were formerly the major killers.

This development was foretold decades ago by the homoeopathic physicians who warned against overindulgence in the vaunted new medicines which were flooding the market. They warned that these substances of increasingly powerful effect, and which were being used with less and less discrimination, were only suppressive in their action and would inevitably cause an increase in chronic disease conditions.

The homoeopathic warnings were ignored, and many physicians to this day remain unaware of the relation-

[54] Arthur L. Herbst, Howard Ulfelder, and David Poskanzer, "Adenocarcinoma of the Vagina: Association of Maternal Stilbestrol Therapy with Tumor Appearance in Young Women," *New England Journal of Medicine* 284 (April 22, 1971), 878–881.

ship between prior medication and the onset of chronic disease.

Another aspect of this problem, to which orthodox medicine is equally inattentive, is the connection between therapeutic procedures and the incidence of mental disease. At present, about one third of the hospital beds in the United States are filled by mental patients.[55] Homoeopathic theory indicates that many of these illnesses are due to powerful drugs administered on incorrect principles; these suppress the physical symptoms and thereby transfer the pathology to the brain.

A statistical investigation of the relationship between prior medication and chronic physical and mental illness would be difficult to conduct, and its results would hardly be free from ambiguity, but facts remain facts even when they cannot be proved to the satisfaction of the medical community (which would have the most to lose from any public recognition of such facts). The least that can be said is that the existence of such a causal relationship is highly probable on theoretical grounds.

It follows logically that the process can only be reversed by altering the whole trend of allopathic pharmacological thought. Medicines must be found which are more specific, more selective, in their effect, and some way must be devised to measure this specific or selective effect. In other words, the homoeopathic alternative must be investigated, since experience has shown that the highly specific indications needed can only be the individualized symptomatic indications used in homoeopathy. Support for this view can be found in the writings of no less an authority than Rene Dubos, who stated not long ago:

---

[55] *Hospitals* XLV (August 1, 1971), Guide Issue, Part II, p. 447.

Most biological, physiological, and biochemical research has been focused so far on the study of the phenomena which are common to all living things. From the point of view of scientific philosophy, the largest achievement of modern biochemistry has been the demonstration of the fundamental *unity* of the chemical processes associated with life. Bacteria, yeasts, liver cells, pigeon muscle, squid nerve fibers, etc., have been selected as objects for biological research not because of their own specific peculiarities but merely for reasons of convenience. The investigator uses these materials for the discovery of general biochemical and physiological laws, not for the identification of components which are peculiar to the organism or the function.

While this so-called fundamental approach has been immensely fruitful for the discovery of the structures and reactions which are *common* to all forms of life, it has almost completely failed to provide information concerning the structures and reactions which determine the *peculiarities* of each organ and function. As a result, the search for metabolic inhibitors has been limited to attempts at interfering with processes ubiquitous in all living beings, for the simple reason that these are the only ones which are known. Powerful metabolic inhibitors have been synthesized on the basis of this knowledge, but in general they lack selectivity. Being directed against fundamental processes, they affect many different biological functions and are therefore likely to exhibit various forms of toxicity which sharply limit their usefulness.

It is obvious that the sharper the selectivity of a biologically active substance, the greater the probability that it will be innocuous for cells and functions other than the one for which it has been designed. In other words, a substance is more likely to be therapeutically useful if it acts almost uniquely against a structure or an activity peculiar to the organism or function to be affected. Unfortunately, the physiological or chemical definition of these specific features and activities is an aspect of biology which is grossly neglected at the present time.[56]

Without being aware of it, Dubos is calling for a homoeopathic approach to the selection of medicines.

[56] In Paul Talalay, ed., *Drugs in Our Society*, pp. 38–39.

Pathological indications are by their very nature too crude to be the basis for a specific therapy, and as long as they continue to be used, the incidence of iatrogenic disease is bound to rise.

*   *   *   *

The time is ripe for those familiar with homoeopathic therapeutic principles to press for their more general acceptance. The public, and some elements of the medical profession, will welcome an assault on the indiscriminate use of broad-spectrum violent medication. They will readily understand and appreciate the homoeopathic stress on constitutional treatment, reinforcement of the patient's inherent recuperative powers, the long-term follow-up of disease, and the prevention of future acute and chronic disease by use of the appropriate procedures when the patient is in health.

There are a number of hurdles, however, in the way of the widespread adoption of this approach to therapeutics. The first, already discussed above, is the inherent opposition between homoeopathic and allopathic principles. This can be surmounted by publishing and disseminating materials which clarify and explain the homoeopathic medical discipline and demonstrate its basis in scientific method.

Behind this theoretical antagonism, however, is a more serious motive for allopathic hostility to homoeopathy. The accusation that homoeopathy is "unscientific" has frequently served only as a cover for this more fundamental factor of hostility.

A sophisticated view of the relations between homoeopathic and allopathic medicine would recognize that the theoretical dispute has economic roots and that doctrinal arguments serve to justify behavior which is in the physician's economic interest. The basic reason for allopathic rejection of homoeopathic principles is that these principles hold the physician to a standard of performance which is intellectually more demanding, and sometimes less economically rewarding, than the ordinary mode of allopathic practice.

We have already shown that the homoeopathic physician must have an intimate knowledge of many hundreds of different drugs, only one of which will suit the particular patient before him. The precise differentiation among diseased states and among medicines is arduous and time-consuming intellectual work.

Homoeopathy has always been plagued by the fundamental requirement that the physician devote substantial time to diagnosis of his patient and selection of the remedy. No technique has yet been devised for bypassing the difficult stages of symptom elucidation and repertorization. Thus homoeopathy could not use the time-saving procedures developed by orthodox medicine, the "broad-spectrum" drugs which in many cases obviate the need for diagnosis, the farming out of certain procedures to para-medical personnel. Homoeopathy cannot be practised on an assembly-line.

On the other hand, all who have had experience with homoeopathy view it as far more effective therapeutically than the method used in orthodox medicine. The time-saving techniques which enhance the physician's income only too often have a deleterious effect on the patient's health.

Today's homoeopathic physician is in a dilemma. He knows that his system of practice is therapeutically sound. At the same time, he finds that he may have to take a reduced income if he is really to be an effective physician. Thus homoeopathy does not appeal to everyone. It is simply too difficult for the ordinary practitioner,

71

too demanding for all but those who, for whatever reason, are willing to make a certain material and personal sacrifice to practice a truly scientific medicine. One of today's foremost homoeopathic physicians has stated the problem succinctly:

Homoeopathy refuses to reveal its secrets to a casual enquirer. The study of an individual in his illness, though fascinating, is sufficiently time-consuming. It caters essentially to the idealistic type of mind which craves for the satisfaction that comes from 'a job well done', and which considers material gains as only incidental. It will suit the hard-working conscientious physician with a philosophical bent of mind which takes readily to the study of the emotional and intellectual sides of man. It will suit a physician who has an individual bent of mind and strong convictions that enable him to swim against the current and even isolate himself from the medical fraternity, if need be. Homoeopathy demands full adherence to its principles if consistent results are to be obtained.

Thus, it will hardly appeal to a physician with a mechanical bent of mind which is so essential for the making of a good surgeon. Persons hankering after 'mass treatments' and 'specifics' will be disillusioned. Physicians who look forward to a life of ease and comfort and who are 'constitutionally averse to work' will abhor the practice of homoeopathy and, if at all they take to it, they will bring little credit either to the Science or to themselves. Although homoeopathy never lets down badly its faithful follower and assures him a reasonable living and standing in the community, the material gains are not such as to satisfy the more ambitious![57]

Homoeopathy will thus appeal to the idealist who is not in the practice of medicine primarily to earn the highest income in the community, but rather to be of service to his fellow man.

[57]Dhawale, *Principles and Practice of Homoeopathy*, Vol. I, pp. 23–24.

At the same time, there are many other positive aspects. The physician knows that his patients are receiving the best care possible. They will probably be sick less frequently, will recover more rapidly, and will lead longer lives. Many will realize that this is due to the efforts of their physician and will reward him with the loyalty and affection which is the hallmark of the relationship between homoeopathic physicians and their patients. At a time when the press and public opinion are increasingly critical of the ordinary practice of orthodox medicine, the homoeopaths continue to retain the full trust and affection of their patients. Once a person has experienced the benefits of homoeopathic treatment, he will usually remain with it throughout his life and will often take extraordinary pains to ensure that he and his family retain access to homoeopathy at a time when the supply of these physicians is still restricted.

Another positive feature of homoeopathy is the intellectual thrill of practising a precise form of medicine. Every case is a new challenge, and every successful prescription vindicates the physician's intellectual and moral qualities. This can be a rare form of satisfaction.

These positive features, however, become evident only after the physician has been in practice for several years. The negative aspects loom most prominently at the outset and undoubtedly discourage many students who would be willing to engage in this form of practice if only it appeared more advantageous economically. Those who persevere through the initial stage of trials and discouragement, until the necessary experience in prescribing is acquired, must necessarily be persons who stand out in the crowd for their qualities of mind and heart and for their willingness to make the extra effort which a scientific form of therapeutics demands.

*B0050 THE LUYTIES REFERENCE HANDBOOK. Compiled from the earlier "Family Doctor" booklet, this new volume retains a nostalgic appearance while presenting valuable information on the homeopathic combinations. Included are a short materia medica, a handy reference to the combinations and a therapeutic index. Useful information for both the physician and layman. An excellent companion to **Luyties Homeopathic Practice** and **The Biochemic Handbook.** $1.25

•B0051 THE BIOCHEMIC HANDBOOK A very useful book to keep on hand. It contains a section on the theory of Biochemistry explained in layman's terms, a section on the use of the various tissue salts and their combinations, a therapeutic index with explanation and a fine repertory. An excellent reference book for both novice and expert. $1.25

•B0052 LUYTIES HOMEOPATHIC PRACTICE Edward L. Perry, M.D. An updated republication of one of the most popular reference books. This is an excellent book for the layman as well as the practicing physician. In addition to its complete therapeutic index, there is a brief materia medica and explanation of the homeopathic theory. Every family should have one of these healing guides. $1.65

*B0053 BIOCHEMISTRY UP-TO-DATE Eric F.W. Powell Ph.D., N.D. This informative book lists and explains the uses of both Schussler's original twelve biochemic salts and thirty more elements used by modern biochemists. Includes a quick reference treatment guide. $2.95

B0054 NATURAL PARENTHOOD Eda J. Leshan. Subtitled "Raising Your Children without a Script," this helpful book is based upon the premiss that children are rugged individualists and no single theory, formula or "script" can instruct a parent in the precise right way to raise children. This book tries to help the parent understand human growth and development so that he can better apply his own wisdom and common sense to the job of child raising. .95

B0055 ACUPUNCTURE, A LAYMAN'S VIEW Lucille Ann Leong. This book explains the traditional Chinese art of treatment by acupuncture and the philosophy upon which it is based. An excellent book for the curious layman who has been both fascinated and confused by the sudden burst of publicity about this ancient medical technique. $1.50

B0056 PLEASE BREAST-FEED YOUR BABY Alice Gerard. A book that answers many of the questions a new mother faces in deciding whether or not to breast-feed her baby. It explains the emotional and physical benefits of breast-feeding to both mother and baby, and deals with the fears the new mother may face. $1.25

B0057 THE NEW AMERICAN MEDICAL DICTIONARY AND HEALTH MANUAL A straightforward translation of medical terms into understandable language. In the words of the author "it is our belief that people are entitled to know as precisely as possible, what physicians mean when they use complicated or esoteric terminology or when they refer to obscure tests and procedures." **$2.25**

*B0058 THE TREATMENT OF CATS BY HOMOEOPATHY K. Sheppard An excellent book for any cat owner. It lists many of the illness and other health problems to which cats are prone, and lists the homeopathic remedy that can be administered safely. It is extremely useful in advising steps that should be taken when a veterinarian is not available. **$2.95**

*B0059 THE TREATMENT OF DOGS BY HOMOEOPATHY by K. Sheppard A companion volume to the one on the treatment of cats. It explains how canine disorders can be safely treated through homeopathic methods, and how to provide relief for the dog when a veterinarian is not available. **$2.95**

*B0060 HOMOEOPATHY FOR THE FIRST-AIDER Dr. Dorothy Shepherd A handy book of homeopathic remedies for situations in which first aid must be administered. Includes suggestions for dealing with pain, aches, bruises, wounds, hemorrhage, burns and scalds, poisons, boils, carbuncles and many more. **$2.95**

*B0061 PROVEN REMEDIES J. H. Oliver N.A.M.H. A collection of common ailments and their homeopathic, herbal, and biochemic treatment, in an easy reference form. **$1.75**

*B0062 BIOCHEMIC PRESCRIBER Eric F. W. Powell Ph.D., N.D. A handy reference guide that explains the use of the twelve tissue salts, and lists alphabetically common symptoms with their homeopathic remedies. **$1.95**

B0063 DR. SCHUESSLER'S BIOCHEMISTRY J.B. Chapman, M.D. edited by J.W. Cogswell, M.D. A complete explanation of Schuessler's twelve tissue salts and their application, written especially for the layman. The author was chosen at the suggestion of Dr. Schuessler himself, and since its original publication it has been a standard work that every person seriously interested in homeopathy should consult. **$11.50**

B0064 THE MOTHERS' MEDICAL ENCYCLOPEDIA Virginia E. Pomeranz M.D. and Dodi Schultz. A complete reference book that any parent will find extremely useful. It defines and explains medical terminology, gives first-aid instructions, and helps a parent understand and help the family physician. **$1.75**

*B0065 THE TWELVE TISSUE REMEDIES Drs. Boericke & Dewey M.D.'s. A very complete book, originally written for the professional but it is very useful for the advanced student. Complete with case histories. **$7.00**

B0066 THE PRINCIPLES AND ART OF CURE BY HOMEOPATH Herbert A. Roberts, M.D. This excellent book deals with the basic principles of homeopathy, and has been used as an official text by The Hahnemann Medical College of Philadelphia. It is certainly a book that the serious student should study. **$9.00**

*B0067 LEADERS IN HOMOEOPATHIC THERAPEUTICS E.B. Nash M.D. This hardbound book treats the more common homeopathic remedies in a modern materia medica for use by the practicing physician and the knowledgeable layman. $4.50

*B0069 REPERTORY TO HOMEOPATHIC MATERIA MEDICA J.D. Kent M.D. A book which deserves the title of "definitive." It is one of the most complete works to aid in the prescription of the correct remedies. Deluxe Edition. $30.00

*B0070 MATERIA MEDICA WITH REPERTORY William Boericke M.D. This is a handy reference book, almost pocketsize and printed on bible thin paper, so that it is small enough to carry yet packed full of information. It has a good description of most homeopathic remedies, their uses, a repertory of the more common symptoms, and many useful indexes. $12.50

*B0072 HOMEOPATHIC MEDICINE Harris L. Coulter. A comprehensive study of the history and theories of homeopathic medicine by one of the country's leading medical historians. A recent work (1972), it answers many questions about the philosophy and method of homeopathic medicine. $1.65

B0073 HOMEOPATHY — MEDICINE OF THE NEW MAN George Vithoulkas. A complete introduction to the Natural System of Medicine. This book outlines the tenets of the long-ignored medical methodology of homeopathy. It includes a good bibliography and listings of homeopathic organizations and societies. $1.25

*B0074 A CLINICAL REPERATORY TO THE DICTIONARY OF MATERIA MEDICA John H. Clarke. Essential for quick and accurate selection of remedies, this book provides the necessary information in an admirably concise manner, making it an indispensable supplement to Dr. Clarke's famous Dictionary. Part One give remedies for many disorders, arranged alphabetically. Part Two deals with Causation. Part Three examines Temperaments, Dispositions, Constitutions and States. Part Four indicates Clinical Relationships. $12.00

B0075 THE BIOCHEMIC SYSTEM OF MEDICINE George W. Carey M.D. edited by Edward L. Perry A.B. M.D. A complete introduction to the Twelve Tissue Salts. This is a textbook which covers theory, application, includes a materia medica and reperatory. Temporarily out of stock. $14.00

*B0076 INTRODUCTION TO THE HOMEOTHERAPEUTICS Drs. W.W. Young, W.P. Baker, and Allen C. Neiswander. A beginner's textbook for physicians interested in the principles and methodology of prescribing for the sick. Valuable to the advanced layman, too. 1974 ed. $15.00

*B0097-8-9 DIVIDED LEGACY Harris L. Coulter. A history of the schism in medical thought, in 3 volumes. Volumes I and II are a study of professional attitudes toward scientific method in medicine, from the time of Hippocrates through the 19th century. Vol. III places this discussion in the context of 19th and early 20th century society, showing how the professional discussion was influenced by socio-economic factors. $17.50 ea.